T0146780

90 Days to
Holistic
Wellness

balancing your BODY, MIND, HEART and SOUL

TRACY MARTORANA

BALBOA.
PRESS

A DIVISION OF HAY HOUSE

Balboa Press books may be ordered through booksellers or by contacting:

Balboa Press
A Division of Hay House
1663 Liberty Drive
Bloomington, IN 47403
www.balboapress.com
1 (877) 407-4847

Because of the dynamic nature of the Internet, any web addresses or
links contained in this book may have changed since publication and
may no longer be valid. The views expressed in this work are solely those
of the author and do not necessarily reflect the views of the publisher,
and the publisher hereby disclaims any responsibility for them.

The author of this book does not dispense medical advice or prescribe the use
of any technique as a form of treatment for physical, emotional, or medical
problems without the advice of a physician, either directly or indirectly. The
intent of the author is only to offer information of a general nature to help
you in your quest for emotional and spiritual well-being. In the event you use
any of the information in this book for yourself, which is your constitutional
right, the author and the publisher assume no responsibility for your actions.

Any people depicted in stock imagery provided by Thinkstock are models,
and such images are being used for illustrative purposes only.
Certain stock imagery © Thinkstock.

Print information available on the last page.

ISBN: 978-1-5043-3002-2 (sc)
ISBN: 978-1-5043-3004-6 (hc)
ISBN: 978-1-5043-3003-9 (e)

Library of Congress Control Number: 2015904427

Balboa Press rev. date: 05/12/2015

Hello. I'm so excited that you have taken the first step in living a more healthy, happy and balanced life! Together, we will identify small steps you can take that will slowly build into dramatic life changes.

Please be sure that you check with your doctor before implementing changes to your diet or physical fitness routine.

■ Table of Contents

■ INTRODUCTION

My name is Tracy Martorana. I am a Nutrition and Wellness Consultant, an Herbalist, a Meditation Instructor, a Mother, Wife, Daughter, Sister and Friend. My passion is to help people get back to the basics of healthy living, in a way that makes them feel fulfilled, happy and healthy. Years ago, I was right where you may be; realizing that my current lifestyle was unfulfilling. I was feeding my body unhealthy, highly processed foods. I made excuses to avoid exercise. And, other than working and raising my daughter, I had few hobbies or interests. Today, while I am far from perfect (thank goodness, perfect is boring), I eat foods that nourish my body, I find ways to bring movement into my day, I meditate, and I find fulfilling work in helping others do the same. In other words, these days I am living my life in a way that makes me feel fulfilled, happy and healthy. Because you are reading this book, I assume you want the same thing. Thank you for allowing me to help you on your journey.

Many people incorrectly correlate healthy living with boring food, a dull life and an overall feeling of deprivation. I think this is because people have forgotten what healthy living really means. The world of technology and convenience has led us into bad habits that leave us feeling unfulfilled, stressed and wore out. We sit way too much and we eat foods that don't nourish the body. We choose zoning out in front of the TV over building relationships with people. We think of healthy eating as a fad diet and exercise as a chore. We don't give our minds a chance to rest, we don't nourish relationships and we don't feed our passions.

Healthy living is exactly the opposite of all of that! Eating real food that nourishes the body gives us the energy to engage in fun activities. Just small amounts of exercise keep us limber and young. Meditation calms our mind and provides us with a sense of wellbeing, self-acceptance and even helps us get a better night's sleep. Engaging our mind allows us to enjoy interests that we can share with others whom we care about.

My goal is to help you take small, actionable steps over the next 3 months, to slowly make changes that will support a healthy, happy and fulfilling life. You might ask, "If these changes are so wonderful, why not jump in and make them all now?" That is a common question and a common mistake that many people make. It all comes down to positive and negative reinforcement.

Let's say today you exercise very little, but a friend has convinced you to run a 5k with her next month. You set out to get ready for the race. You get yourself a new pair of sneakers, put them on and jog for 30 minutes. Whew, it almost killed you, but you did it! You are so proud of yourself for taking this step to get ready for the race. Tomorrow rolls around and you realize you can barely walk. Your whole body aches from the abnormal amount of exercise you put it through. The next day comes. Oh no, day 2 is even worse as the lactic acid has caused every muscle to tighten and ache even more than yesterday. Day 3...things are starting to loosen up, but walking still hurts and the thought of climbing stairs still makes you wince. You think maybe you should try to run again if you really want to do this 5k, but your ankles are still tight and maybe even a little swollen. You decide this pain just isn't worth it. You call your friend and say, sorry – I just can't run...it hurts too much. The negative reinforcement won.

You started off with great intentions, but simply took on too much, too fast. The result wasn't a positive one...you suffered severe pain. This result does not reinforce the action you wanted to take. However, if you slowed things down...started with walking 30 minutes, then after a couple days you add in jogging a few minutes throughout a 30 minute walk. You would add more minutes of jogging each week, building your fitness level slowly, without pain. Instead of pain, you would have the positive reinforcement of accomplishment, of day after day being able to move toward your goal. You would feel the exhilaration of the physical exercise without the pain. You would feel positive feelings about the steps you are taking and you would be much more likely to continue with these actions and slowly reach the goal you have in mind. You would obtain the benefits of your healthy actions.

This is why New Year Resolutions rarely work. People bite off too much all at once and receive some sort of negative feedback that stops them from continuing on the path they desire. They give up. Face it, negative reinforcement really works...often better than positive reinforcement. That is why it is so important to keep changes small and minimize these negative effects.

With this book, I am going to walk you through small changes you can make every week to slowly move in the direction of holistic wellness. We will build on these changes week over week. If you find you have a lot of work to do on any given subject, stay on the step for a couple of weeks to slowly make improvements. Then, when you are ready, you can move on to the next step. I set the book up for 90 days, but for many people it takes longer. And truthfully, after 90 days, you will still have work to do. I suggest that when you finish the book, you revisit it again, and take each improvement to the next level. We can all find ways to continuously improve our lifestyle choices, even me (and I wrote the book)!

And that is exactly how I've made so many healthy changes myself. Years ago, it was not unusual for my dinner to consist of Pop-tarts and Pepsi. Once I decided I wasn't happy with how I felt every day, I knew I needed to make some changes. Like many others, I would jump into it with both feet...and I would fail. I would try again, completely transforming my eating habits. I would try to eat nothing but healthy foods that I didn't even like, just because that was what someone told me healthy eating was. I would set my alarm and get up early to walk on the treadmill. And time after time, I would end up right back where I started or even worse off! Why? Because I didn't care much for salads, I was not a morning person and I hated the treadmill. I would rebound from these failures by grabbing a candy bar, refusing to exercise at all and wallowing in self-loathing. Eventually I realized that making these big sweeping changes didn't work for me. I essentially gave up, until I realized I didn't have to make such severe changes and they didn't have to be all at once. I didn't have this book to follow back then, so my efforts were haphazard and therefore it took me a lot longer that it needed to. But eventually, change after change, I slowly moved baby step by baby step from Pop-tarts and Pepsi to quinoa and roasted vegetables. You can make changes too! Just remember to keep the changes small and build on them over and over, until soon you will find you are living the life you desire...healthy, happy and balanced.

Note:

Right off, I want to warn you...the changes we are making are not large and they are not hard. However because we are making a series of these small changes, you do have to be committed. Life is all about priorities, and sadly, many of us do not live our lives in line with our priorities. It is so easy to procrastinate or ignore what you know is good for you. So as you start this journey, I ask you to take a moment and pledge to yourself that your health, your well-being and your happiness are all priorities to you and you will treat them as such. We only have one ride on this carousel (that we know of for sure), and only one body to do it in. Together, let's do all we can to be sure our body, mind, heart and soul can sustain the many years of bliss we fully intend on enjoying!

■ HOLISTIC WELLNESS

Holistic Wellness is more than just healthy eating...

As a Nutrition and Wellness consultant and an herbalist, I believe food is medicine. Good nutrition and living close to the earth are important first steps in disease prevention and in living a healthy, holistic lifestyle.

But there is more to it than just nutrition. Holistic Wellness means to live in a way that nurtures all aspects of your being. The following graphic illustrates this example.

body
- Nutrition
- Exercise
- Personal Care

heart
- Time with Family
- Friends
- Charity

mind
- Lifetime Learning
- Work
- Environmental Care

soul
- Spirituality
- Religion
- Journaling
- Time in Nature

Making small changes in your behaviors regarding these aspects of yourself, is the most sustainable way to make big changes in your lifestyle. You make a small change this week, another small change next week, then another and another... Before you realize it, you are living a much healthier and happier life.

One thing to note, this book doesn't directly address vices. If you do an honest assessment of your lifestyle, you might identify some vices you would do better without. Maybe you drink a little more than you should, you smoke, you gamble too much, you watch too much TV...the list could go on. I find that when it comes to changing lifestyle choices, vices are the things people are most attached too. They are painful to quit, often even part of our identity. Therefore, the act of giving up a vice is often riddled with negative reinforcement such as withdrawal and negative attitudes from friends that share the vice with you.

Because of the negative reinforcement that comes along with giving up vices, it is often better to start with focus on adding positive habits or doing something new versus stopping a habit. Eventually, all the positive changes will likely inspire you to take the deep dive into quitting a bad habit. Also, it is difficult to work giving up vices into this format of change, since everyone's vices are so different.

I'm not suggesting you *ignore* your bad habits....just allow yourself to release them naturally! As your lifestyle becomes healthier, you will find that vices slowly decrease. However, you may find that you have a habit that you need or want to address now. For this I would suggest that you still start slow. Remember, negative reinforcement works, so you must try to minimize it while creating some positive effects. For example...

If you want to quit smoking, make positive changes that will indirectly affect your smoking habits. Going to bed ½ hour earlier every day may be the catalyst for skipping that last cigarette of the night. Jogging or walking in the morning may help you move your first cigarette until later in the morning. Meeting with a non-smoking friend at a smoke-free restaurant for lunch may help you cut out a lunchtime cigarette. The focus here is not directly on reducing smoking...it is about making positive changes in other areas of your life, that happen to affect your smoking habit.

Are you ready to get started? First things first. You are going to need to keep track of the changes you will be making. The easiest way to do this is with Appendix 1, the 90 Day Goal List. You can simply make a copy of the page in this book, or better yet; you can print a full sized copy directly from my website:

http://www.holisticwellnesswithtracy.com/90-days-to-holistic-wellness-goal-list.html

Now, let's get started!

■ Week #1: Nutrition - Focus on Fruits & Vegetables

I'm starting with this because it's the top "issue" for the majority of my clients. We all know that a healthy diet should contain lots of fruits and veggies, however most people I know do not meet the USDA recommendations for their daily intake. I believe the main reason for this is that our busy lifestyles have led to a cooking style that does not focus on fresh food. The typical vegetables served up with dinner are often just microwaved frozen chunks or an emptied can, presented with no pizzazz and little flavor or texture. Is that true for you as well?

With just a little bit of creativity, you can serve up delicious vegetable dishes!

Let's talk a little about how many vegetables & fruits are enough. The USDA now uses the ChooseMyPlate graphic to describe daily intake of food groups. You can find this graphic and other information provide by the U.S. Department of Agriculture or USDA at http://www.choosemyplate.gov.

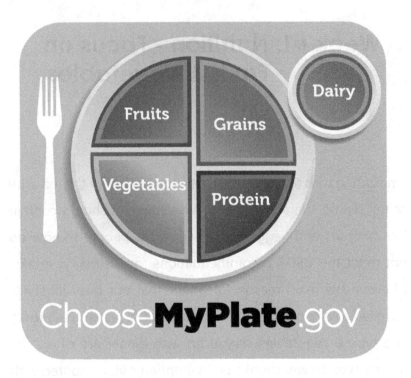

For many people, this graphic makes meal planning easier. However, it has its drawbacks. It can be difficult to use if you don't eat regular meals every day and it gives no guidelines about snacks.

When it comes down to how many servings of fruits and vegetables you should eat per day (meals and snacks), I suggest that for the average person, 2-4 servings of fruits and 3-5 servings of vegetables per day would be appropriate. Note that while fruits and vegetables are often grouped together into one food group, they are not interchangeable. Eating 9 servings of fruit per day would not be a healthy option. This is because fruits tend to be quite high in sugar; and fruits and vegetables have different vitamin profiles, making both important. When it comes to eating fruits and vegetables I have 2 suggestions:

1) Eat more vegetables than fruit.
2) Variety really is the spice of life. Yes it prevents boredom, but it is also the best way to get the variety of vitamins and minerals your body needs.

If you are not a big veggie eater, this can seem like a lot, I know! Don't let this overwhelm you. Remember, you don't have to do it all today! Let's break it down.

First, let's start by looking at what a serving size is:

A typical serving size of a fruit is about 1 cup cubed fresh fruit, ½ cup dried fruit or 1 cup fruit juice. Examples of this would be 1 small orange, ½ a grapefruit, 2 plums, ¼ cup raisins.

A typical serving size of a vegetable is 2 cups leafy vegetable, 1 cup others and 1 cup vegetable juice. Examples of this would be 2 cups raw spinach, 1 cup steamed broccoli or cauliflower, 1 large sweet potato.

Check out the USDA website for further information regarding the MyPlate graphic, food groups and serving sizes. There is a lot of good, up to date information there.

http://www.choosemyplate.gov/food-groups/

Second, take a moment to think about what you typically eat. How many fruits and vegetables do you eat on a typical day? It may be helpful to use the Food Tracker provided as Appendix 2 or write out everything you ate for the last couple of days to give yourself a realistic view of your eating habits (be sure to accurately assess serving sizes). Make a copy of Appendix 2 or print it directly from my website at:

http://www.holisticwellnesswithtracy.com/90-days-to-holistic-wellness-goal-list.html

In my experience, people grossly over estimate their ingestion of healthy foods such as fruits and vegetables.

Because this is such an important item, I would recommend that if you discover you are far away from meeting the USDA guidelines, you may want to consider spending a couple of weeks on this step before moving on, to slowly work on adding more fruits and veggies into your diet. Add 1 additional daily serving this week, and then 1 more daily serving next week. (Another option would be to add 1 daily serving this week and revisit this week's action later in the 90 day process, by adding additional repeat weeks in-between others). Meeting the USDA minimum requirement is very important, so make this change a priority! But remember, you are more likely to stick with the changes if you make them slowly. You may not be ready to fully meet the USDA recommendation for weeks or months...just make steps to move in that direction now. Remember, change is an ongoing process.

Ideas for adding more fruits &vegetables to your diet:

- Start your day with a piece of fruit for breakfast. I love to eat ½ grapefruit with breakfast. If you eat on the go, a banana, apple or grapes make great travel foods.
- "I should've had a V8". Remember that commercial? Have a serving of vegetable juice as a morning snack. V8 has a low-sodium, spicy blend that's pretty tasty.

Add a little dab of horseradish and a stick of celery and you have a virgin Bloody Mary! Or if you are feeling real adventurous, get a juicer and make your own!

- Add Green Leaf lettuce and a couple slices of tomato to your sandwich. Or, get more adventurous and add roasted red peppers, onion, and cucumbers.

- Have a cup of vegetable soup for lunch (look for a low sodium version or make a big batch of soup from scratch).

- Make a veggie omelet for Sunday breakfast – fill it up with every vegetable you love. I like mine with broccoli, bell pepper, onion, mushrooms and a sprinkle of cheese.

- Start dinner with a side salad. Iceburg is good, but other lettuces are so much better. Include greens like spinach, romaine and arugula. Look for prewashed, bagged salad greens to speed up dinner preparation. Experiment!

- Instead of a soda, grab an orange juice.

- Munch on raw veggies as an afternoon snack. Bored already, thinking of nothing but carrot sticks? Include pea pods, green beans, cauliflower, grape tomatoes, celery, bell peppers, even asparagus! Dip them in a yummy flavored hummus. Have these all prepped and ready to eat in your refrigerator for easy snacking all week long.

- Fill half your plate with veggies. Beware, steamed gets boring – roast and grill your veggies for better flavor! Short on time? Look for pre-chopped veggies in your produce department. They cost a tad more, but they can be quite the time saver. Visit my blog for simple recipe ideas: **http://www.holisticwellnesswithtracy. com/blog/category/recipes**

- Pizza for dinner? You can do better than just pepperoni! Veggies make delicious toppings!

- Have a veggie entrée like grilled eggplant parmesan or Mediterranean stuffed portabella mushrooms.

- Make salad for dinner. Imagine a beautiful green salad with red bell peppers, cauliflower, yellow tomatoes and ½ a sliced chicken breast...dressed with a homemade lemon-mustard dressing and sprinkled with sunflower seeds.

- Fruit for dessert. Strawberries macerated with a small sprinkle of sugar and a splash of red wine vinegar (trust me!)

Note:

Don't overdue on the fruits. Many people find it easier to add more fruits to their diets, but too many fruits can lead to increased sugar/calories. Stick with one serving of fruit for every two servings of vegetables.

Now comes the part that leads to actually changing something:

Come up with a plan for adding more fruits and vegetables to your diet. What are you going to add and when? Take a moment to think this through then decide and write it down. Keep it simple. Examples: "Eat a piece of fruit for breakfast every day this week", "Have vegetable soup for lunch weekdays and a salad with dinner on weekends". "I will snack on 1 serving of raw vegetables every afternoon", "I will roast a variety of vegetables on Sunday to easily fill half my plate with them for every weeknight meal". Make it specific enough that you can plan it and track your activity. If you just vaguely say your goal is to eat another serving of vegetables every day, you aren't likely to do it. You need a specific plan to actually follow through on. Enter this into your goal tracker for week 1.

Go shopping and stock your kitchen. Prep what you can so it's ready and waiting, making it as easy as possible to include these foods (if you want a snack and the produce still needs to be washed and chopped, you are more likely to go for another option). Leave a fruit bowl on the kitchen table. Pack lunches the night before so you don't rush out of the house without it. Experiment with different foods, different cooking methods and different spices. There are many wonderful and delicious ways to prepare veggies. If you find your food choices boring, you can't blame it on the "healthy" food...you can only blame it on the preparation.

Need help planning out meals & making your shopping list? Print the Meal Planning_Shopping List tool from appendix 3 or print from my website:

http://www.holisticwellnesswithtracy.com/90-days-to-holistic-wellness-goal-list.html

Note:

If you are meeting the USDA recommendations, you could move on to the next chapter, or you could consider if there are still any changes you could make here. If you eat pretty much the same few fruits and vegetables, spend this week experimenting with some new produce. If you tend to douse your salads with high fat dressings try homemade vinaigrettes. Then carry these new changes with you into the future.

■ Week #2: Fitness - Just Move

Many of us spend too much time sitting. We watch too much TV, we sit at the computer and we sit in the car or on the train.

It is recommended that we get 150 minutes of moderate exercise a week. If you do the math, that's 30 minutes/5 times a week. That can be difficult to manage in our busy world. I know, that statement sounds a bit like an oxymoron; we are so busy we don't have time to move? For many of us, that seems to be the case. We don't have labor intensive jobs and we live in communities where walking or biking just isn't a viable option.

Why do we care so much about exercise? We all know that exercise can help control weight, but did you know it is also a mood enhancer, helps prevent several diseases, increases energy levels, helps you sleep better and even improves your sex life? If you want to read more about these benefits, check out: http://www.mayoclinic.org/healthy-living/fitness/in-depth/exercise/art-20048389.

Hopefully you agree that regular exercise is beneficial for a happy and healthy life. If you doubt this for even a moment, consider how it feels having the strength to lift a bag of groceries, the range of motion to pick something up off the floor and the energy to play with your dog versus feeling weak, stiff and fatigued. Which scenario feels best to you? The goal of exercise is not to make you look like a supermodel or to prep you for the cover of GQ...it is to make you comfortable in your body, feeling energetic and healthy.

If you don't already get the amount of exercise recommended, then it's best to start with increasing your exercise level just a small amount. Now, I can already hear many of you chiming in "I really don't have the time!" I can assure you, while I make the same excuses some days, it really just isn't true. There are people far busier than us, who manage to exercise every day. How? They make it a priority.

Take a good, hard, honest look at the activity you get every week. Are you getting less than 30 minutes / 5 days a week? Since this is most likely the case, this week we will focus on increasing your movement. You can do this in several different ways. Keep in mind that the exercise does not have to occur in one 30 minute session. It can easily be broken down into three 10 minute sessions, if that fits your lifestyle and schedule better.

Ideas for adding more exercise to your day...even just 10 minutes:

- Start your day with a 10 minute walk around your neighborhood.
- If you work in a large building, use the bathroom that is furthest away.
- Make a habit of parking your car far away from your destination.
- Walk during your lunch break.
- Go for an evening walk after dinner with a spouse/child/neighbor.
- Go for a bike ride.
- Play kickball with your kids/grandkids/nieces/nephews.
- Instead of meeting a friend for a drink, meet them for a walk.
- Do some stretching and/or crunches while watching TV.
- Carefully stretch for 5 minutes after showering in the morning. Then do a few lunges to work your legs.
- Rather than calling or sending an email to a coworker, get up and walk to their desk.

- Wear a pedometer to measure your steps. Every day, aim for more steps than the previous day and don't sit down for the evening until you've done it!
- Take your dog outside to play fetch.

This week, in addition to including your additional daily serving of veggies, you will add a new change that involves adding 10 minutes of activity to your daily routine. Consider what would work best for you. What time of the day would be easiest for you? Will you have to get up a few minutes earlier or call a friend to plan evening walks? Determine how you can most successfully add additional activity into your day and then add it to your goal tracker sheet for week 2. Remember, be specific....examples: "I will walk 10 minutes at lunch during the week, and take a 20 minute bike ride on Sunday", "I will walk the dog around the block every day before I shower".

Use the tracker forms to log your progress. You can copy these tools from the appendix or print it directly from my website at: http://www.holisticwellnesswithtracy.com/90-days-to-holistic-wellness-goal-list.html

Note:

If you are already meeting or exceeding the 150 minutes/week recommendation, consider mixing things up by trying something new!

■ Week #3: Meditation

For many people, meditation is a scary word. When you think of meditation, do you think of a monk sitting like a pretzel for hours on end? Or do you think it's only for someone with hours of spare time? Meditation, in its simplest definition, is just mindfulness. It is about being present in the moment. It's about taking some time to let your mind be quiet. It's about giving your left brain a mundane focus so your right brain has time to shine.

How often do you simply sit in silence? In this day and age, with Facebook, smart phones, kindles and our perpetual to-do lists, we rarely just sit...disconnected from the world. We don't take the time to learn who we are when we aren't interacting with others or reading what others think. Technology can be wonderful, but it has robbed us of this gift. Meditation is the simplest way for you to enjoy silence, experience peace and to connect with yourself and the divine (because really, they are one and the same). For most of us, the answer to the question "how often do you simply sit in silence?" is rarely or never. Because of this, we often find ourselves stressed, frantic, and lost in judgment... our judgment of others and our worries of how others are judging us. Meditation is one sure-fire way to let go of the mental clutter and chaos, to let go of judgment, to get to know and love ourselves for who we really are.

If you have never tried meditation before or weren't impressed with it before, let go of your preconceived judgments. Mediation is simple, natural and there are many easy ways to include meditation in your day. While I have heard several teachers say that you *need* to meditate 20 minutes, twice a day. That is simply not a viable option for most people, especially if you are new to meditation. And, more importantly, it just isn't true. Just one minute can bring a sense of calmness....more is nice, but there is nothing wrong with starting small, it's how we do things here, right? Let's talk a little more about meditation.

In my mind, meditation is one of the single most important things you can do to live your life from a place of holistic wellness (along with eating your vegetables). Why? Meditation affects every aspect of your being. In the beginning of the book I shared a 2x2 square depicting Holistic Wellness. Below is the same grid, but this time it's filled with benefits of meditation.

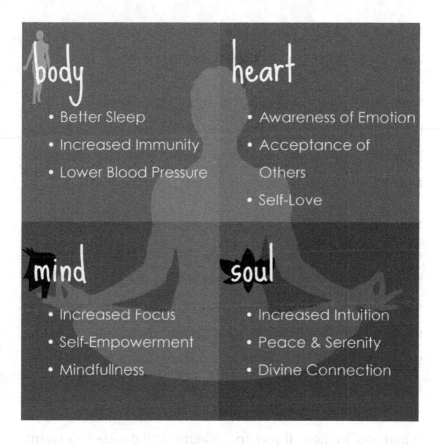

body
- Better Sleep
- Increased Immunity
- Lower Blood Pressure

heart
- Awareness of Emotion
- Acceptance of Others
- Self-Love

mind
- Increased Focus
- Self-Empowerment
- Mindfullness

soul
- Increased Intuition
- Peace & Serenity
- Divine Connection

A picture (or graphic) is worth a thousand words! So, now that you understand the many, many benefits of meditation, I think you will agree that it's worth including this in your daily life!

To clarify, let's discuss meditation just a little more and then I will present ideas for the practice of meditation.

Meditation can be done anywhere. Sometimes you may choose to sit quietly with your eyes closed, other times you may be standing in line somewhere with your eyes open.

Meditation can be done while being still, or it may be done while walking, jogging or hula-hooping.

Meditation is not a religious practice, unless you want it to be. It can be done in connection with a religious ceremony, in tandem with prayer; or simply used as a tool for relaxation and self-discovery.

This week, in addition to your increase in fruits and vegetables and 10 minutes of walking (or other exercise), I request that you add in a daily meditation. I'm not talking about a long, time consuming practice...just 1-2 minutes a day. Below are several suggestions. They aren't complicated (I promise), but they are surprisingly beneficial. Look at my suggestions and pick one and do it every day, or pick a different one each day to try out several and see what works best for you. The important thing is that you do them. If you do 2 minutes and decided you want to keep going for another few minutes, feel free...sometimes once you start, you realize how good it can feel!

Simple Meditation Ideas (remember, meditation = mindfulness):

- Close your eyes and take 5-10 slow deep breaths. Concentrate fully on your breath. Hear your breath, feel your chest expand in all directions, feel your breath on your throat and nostrils.

- While doing anything (washing your hands, brushing your teeth, pulling weeds), focus completely on what you are doing. Be completely mindful, using all the senses involved; focus on the smell, the feel, the look, the sound, the taste.

- No matter where you are, pick one sense and focus on it.
  - o Close your eyes and spend 1 minute picking out every different sound you can hear.
  - o Look around you and mentally describe everything you see, in detail.
  - o Close your eyes and note every sensation you can feel in your body.

- Hula-hoop. This takes a fair amount of mindful concentration!

- Another breathing option; with your eyes open or closed, work to slow your exhalation. Breathe in for a count of 4 and then slowly exhale for a count of 8. You must maintain concentration and control to physically slow down the exhalation.

- Just sit in silence...no checking the phone, no reading, no watching TV.

During all of these exercises, thoughts are likely to pop into your mind. Simply let the thoughts pass, and bring your attention back to what you are focusing on, whether it's your breath, a sound, a sensation or just the feelings of being. It will get easier with practice!

Decide when, where and how you will meditate. If your plan requires any preparation (finding relaxing music or asking family members to allow you a few minutes of private time), take care of that now. Record your specific goal on the tracker sheet(s) and enjoy this new activity.

Note:

If you already meditate regularly, take this week to expand your practice. Practice longer or more often; or, try a new form of meditation that you don't normally use.

If you are interested in trying a guided meditation, visit:

http://www.holisticwellnesswithtracy.com/gifts-from-me-to-you.html

■ Week #4: Decrease Chemical Exposure

In our daily lives, we are exposed to chemicals all the time. Many of these can make us sick, from allergies to cancer. We come into contact with chemicals in many different ways. We apply them to our bodies in creams and perfumes, we breathe them while cleaning or driving in traffic, and we ingest them in our food, from fertilizers to flavor enhancing additives. Everywhere we turn, we are bombarded with chemicals.

In the effort to decrease our exposure to chemicals, many of us spend lots of money on organic foods...all in the effort of avoid pesticides and chemical fertilizers. This is a great way to decrease chemical exposure; however, there are cheaper and equally important places you should look to decrease your chemical exposure. Start by taking a look at your cleaning products.

Many household cleaners are full of chemicals that you really don't want on your skin, in your lungs or in your food. Yes, I say in your food because the cleaners you spray all over your kitchen surely end up in your food as well! Even many of the cleaners marketed as "green" are still filled with things you don't want to be in contact with and they are often quite expensive.

Here are some better options for cleaning your house in order to decrease your exposure to toxic chemicals.

My number one favorite cleaning ingredient is **vinegar**. I use this for everything! Next time you are in the grocery store, pick up a big gallon jug of white vinegar. The store brand is fine, no need to go fancy. For a couple bucks, you have a huge container of cleaning product! Many people worry about the smell...and yes, it does remind me a little bit of coloring Easter eggs while I'm cleaning. However, when vinegar dries, it leaves behind NO SMELL. Real clean has no smell. But, if you want to add a little freshness to the air after cleaning, add a drop of **lemon essential oil** to a damp rag and wipe it over your kitchen counters, your refrigerator, or any surface area you want to freshen up. If lemon isn't the smell you are looking for, there are plenty others – orange, pine, cinnamon. Just be sure the essential oil you use is ingestible (many are not).

So you have the vinegar, now what? Fill an old spray bottle (or buy a new one) almost to the top with vinegar, add just a drop or two of dish soap, a splash of water and you have a great all-purpose cleaner. You can even skip the dish soap if you want. I use this for my kitchen counters, my stove top, my refrigerator, my cutting boards, my toilets and sinks, mirrors, windows and even my floors.

For the tub, just sprinkle the tub with **baking soda** and then spray down with vinegar. The bubbling reaction and the grittiness of the baking soda provide a scratch free/scrubbing bubbles sort of action that is perfect for getting off that stubborn soap scum.

Getting ready to dust your wood furniture? Put away your can of Pledge or Endust and simply take a rag, add a couple drops of **olive oil** and off you go. If you want to jazz it up, add a drop of lemon or orange essential oil, but it's certainly not necessary!

Is your wooden cutting board stained up and a little nasty? You have to be very careful what you spray on your cutting board because it soaks in! A simple way to clean a stain is to sprinkle some **salt** on it, add a little **lemon juice** and scrub. If you are using a real lemon, toss it in your garbage disposal to freshen that up while you're at it!

Need to polish up some silver? Use a paste of vinegar and baking soda. This will also work for bronze and copper and is much better than the chemical tarnish removers that require gloves!!

Speaking of copper – do you have copper bottom pans? Apply a coat of ketchup or tomato sauce to the copper and let it sit for 5-10 minutes, and then wash it off. The acid in the tomatoes removed the tarnish from the copper – brilliant!

After all this cleaning, your house probably just smells clean... like nothing. Before you even consider reaching for a can of air freshener, think for a moment about what is in that can. Before you spray those chemicals into the air you breathe, consider how easy it would be to make your own air-freshener. How? Keep reading....

If you have a small spray bottle, simply add a splash of vodka, a few drops of essential oils and fill with water. Shake and spray. Don't have any vodka? Use real vanilla extract – but beware not to spray too close to fabric as it will discolor it.

Another option of smelling up your home (in a good way) is to take a tart warmer, and instead of adding a wax tart, just add water and a drop or two of essential oils or make your own stovetop potpourri by filling a saucepan with water and adding some good smelling spices like cinnamon and cloves along with the peel of an orange or lemon.

You can also reduce chemical exposure by replacing your scented lotions and perfumes with unscented. If you want a scent, add a drop of good essential oil.

While you are enjoying that extra vegetable serving, 10 minutes of exercise and a couple minutes of daily meditation, consider what change you want to make this week to decrease your chemical exposure. Some ideas....

- Replace your all-purpose cleaner for a spray bottle of vinegar.
- Refer to **http//static.foodnews.org/pdf/EWG-shoppers-guide.pdf** for a list of produce that you should consider purchasing organic and which are not worth the extra cost.
- Dump/recycle any bottles of air freshener you have and replace with a more natural version, like what is listed above.
- Invest in some houseplants. Spider plants, English Ivy, Aloe, Reed Palm and Peace Lilies are known for their air-cleaning properties.
- Replace plastic (PVC) items in your house.

- Use glass food storage containers.
- Use unscented toiletries.
- Replace fabric softener and other smelly products with essential oils. (white vinegar and essential oils makes a great fabric softener)

Okay – get out your goal tracker sheet and commit to one of these things. This is an easy, quick commitment this week, but it still has to be specific! Example: I will buy organic apples this week" or "I will buy a spray bottle and vinegar when I go grocery shopping on Sunday and place next to the sink for daily use". And don't forget to keep up with your previous goals! You are doing great! The extra vegetable serving should be habit by now....you probably don't even think of it as an "extra" serving anymore, the exercise should be feeling good, but not cramping you for time, and those few minutes of meditation probably feel like a gift of peace and calm.

Note:

If you already make your own cleaning products, buy only organic and overall feel you have no chemical exposure; consider your work environment, help a friend clean up their space, teach a class on making cleaning products, give house plants to friends. Or, repeat a previous week – add another vegetable, walk for 15 minutes or expand your meditation.

■ Week #5: Community Service, Charity

"No one has ever become poor by giving."

— <u>Anne Frank</u>, <u>*diary of Anne Frank*</u>

Being of service is one of the most uplifting things you can do for yourself. Wait, did I just say "yourself"? You thought being of service was about others???

I'm being funny, but I'm also serious. Okay, I know...now I'm talking out of both sides of my mouth, which is always difficult to understand! Let me explain what I mean.

Service work is beneficial to everyone involved. Obviously those benefitting from your work are, well...benefitting. But, what about you? How are you benefitting? Doing charity work and/or supporting your community in some way, is personally fulfilling. Just spending a couple hours working for a charity can increase your overall sense of worth and happiness.

What I'm saying is that the concept of altruism is a lie! Altruism means doing something good with no benefit to you. However, it is impossible to do something good for someone without a benefit to you. That benefit might not be material, but you will always get a benefit!

We enter into the second month of change by focusing on others. If you are using the tracker form I included as part of this book, you will notice that last week you really only had to make the effort once, and you reap the benefit for multiple days. I did this on purpose so that so that you don't get bombarded with change after change that you have to engage daily. This week is similar in that it doesn't have to be a daily activity, but it can be. It's really up to you.

This week you are still eating that extra vegetable serving every day, getting at least 10 minutes of light exercise, spending a few minutes practicing mindfulness and you've made a change in your home that is lessening your chemical exposure. So now, what will you do for others (and ultimately yourself)?

I am listing some ideas below, but there are so many others! It all depends on what is important to you. Also, keep in mind that physically getting out and helping is more fulfilling than just writing a check...but do what works best for you.

Ideas for charity work:

- Join your local Rotary or other service club. These clubs provide many opportunities to help out. If you can't join, just contact them to see how you can support them.
- Help out at your local soup kitchen or homeless shelter.
- Clean out your closets and donate gently used clothes to a shelter or other charity.
- Volunteer to play with animals at an animal shelter.
- Ask a local church if they have elderly members that could use help cleaning, cooking or taking care of their yard.
- Volunteer to hold babies at a near-by hospital. There are often babies in ICU that can't go home yet and whose families can't be there often enough.
- Sign up for regular paycheck deductions for charities such as The United Way, The American Heart Association, The American Cancer Society, Audubon, Charity Water or any other charity that speaks to you. I am not endorsing any of these charities, do your

research and find a charity that you believe in, trust and desire to support.

- Put $1 a day into your own "do nice things" fund. Use this money to buy a stranger's coffee, over tip a waiter, or to give to the homeless person you see on the street. The purpose is to create your own random acts of kindness fund.
- Become a big brother or big sister.
- Stop by a nursing home to visit someone that doesn't get many visitors.

Once again, specifically choose how you would like to contribute to society, enter it in your goal worksheet and do whatever you need to do to prepare to make that happen. You may need to call a local charity group to get more info, you may need to arrange paycheck deductions or schedule time to help out somewhere. Resist the urge to write down a goal and tell yourself you will make the calls or do the preparation later – because procrastination often leads to failure to fulfill your goal.

Note:

If you are already involved in charity work, consider doing a little more or try helping out in a different way. Or, work to convince a family member or friend to join you in service.

■ Week #6: Nutrition - Whole Grains & Processed Foods

This week, we return to review our diets. We've already looked at adding more fruits & vegetables to the diet, but that's only half the plate! Remember this picture from week 1?

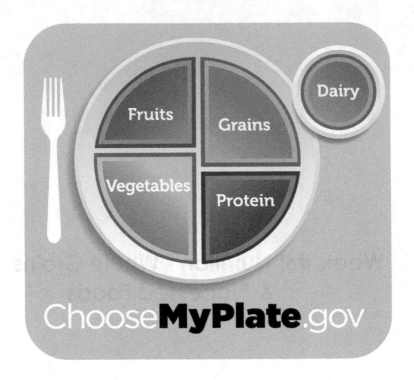

According to ChooseMyPlate.gov, more than a quarter of each meal should be grains. If you remember the old food pyramid, it suggested 6-11 servings of grains a day. The exact number of servings isn't the most pressing issue here (although most people overeat from this food group). The most important thing, not really emphasized in either of these tools, is that at least half of your grains should be whole grains.

Unfortunately, many people gravitate toward refined grains (think white bread and white rice). However, increasing your intake of whole grains has many health benefits. Whole grains have been linked to increased cardiovascular health and decreased risk of diabetes. If you already have high cholesterol, high blood pressure or diabetes, increasing the whole grains in your diet can help you manage and counter these health issues. Whole grains equal high fiber, which is beneficial for digestive health too!

Take a moment to consider your diet and honestly evaluate how many servings of grains you eat in a day, and how many of those are whole grains. Keep in mind what a serving of grains is: 1 slice of bread, ½ bagel, ½ cup pasta or rice, ½ cup cooked cereal, 1 cup cold cereal, or 3-4 crackers. Just a thought regarding pasta; how many servings were on your last plate of pasta?? Appendix 2: Food Tracker may help you with this evaluation.

Next, I want to talk to you briefly about that last quarter of the plate – protein. In the USA, and in most developed countries, ingesting adequate protein is not an issue. In fact, most Americans consume much more than the USDA recommended guidelines. Rarely have I had to advise a client to eat more protein. I have certainly advised people to make better protein choices, but to eat more? No. By better protein choices I mean leaner cuts of meat (vs high fat / processed meats), eggs, nuts, beans, peanut butter, tofu and veggies such as broccoli and spinach. The average adult only requires 46-56 g of protein (less for women than men, more if you are very active vs sedentary). All of the USDA recommendations can be found at: http://www.cnpp.usda.gov/sites/default/files/dietary_guidelines_for_americans/PolicyDoc.pdf

Meeting this requirement is not difficult to do, simply by eating a few (2-3) healthy protein choices a day. Animal products contain more protein than vegetables, but if you are eating your suggested 3-5 servings of vegetables plus some dairy (or dairy alternatives), you are well on your way to meeting your daily protein intake without even purposefully eating "protein foods".

One more topic for this chapter; I would like to take this moment to mention processed foods. We are busy people... it's easy to forget about cooking whole foods and we tend to turn to prepackaged mixes and fast food. You will find however, that as you make healthy protein choices, increase your whole grains and increase your fruit and vegetable intake, the amount of processed foods you eat will slowly decrease. But to help matters along, it is always good to stop and think before buying and preparing any food that comes in a box or a can and has a long ingredient list. You don't need to forgo packaged food products completely...simply be aware of what you are buying. Whenever possible, substitute real, whole foods, for packages. This may mean making plain brown rice and flavoring it yourself with onion, garlic and herbs...find some recipes, play around...make bigger batches to eat over several nights. With a little planning and preparation, you can avoid many processed foods.

You are probably wondering already what goals I am getting ready to ask you to make. This week, there are several options depending on what you think will most benefit you. I suggest taking a minute to honestly contemplate your diet. Yes, I said honestly. Living in denial certainly won't help you any here! Do you eat too many carbohydrates (grains)? Do you eat mostly white/refined grains? Do you eat way too much protein or simply choose high fat or highly processed meats (ham, salami, high fat cuts of beef or pork, sandwich meat)? Is your grocery cart often fill with a lot of prepackaged foods?

Pick the one area you think will make the biggest (or easiest) impact on your diet and set a goal around that. Here are a few suggestions:

Goal: Decrease overall carbohydrate intake. Increase whole grains:

- Continue to increase vegetable consumption. (The more veg you eat, the less carbohydrates you will eat)
- Eat oatmeal for breakfast.
- Substitute whole grain pasta for your white pasta.
- Use brown rice instead of white.

- If you already eat a healthy number of carbohydrates and many are whole grain, consider trying a new grain every week, such as quinoa, farro, barley, amaranth, bulgur.

Goal: Eat healthier proteins:

- Replace high fat / processed foods with leaner cuts (pork chops, chicken breasts, fish) or other forms of proteins (tofu, seitan) and increase vegetable intake.
- Watch portion sizes. A serving of meat is 3-4 oz. Consider this before you order a 16 oz steak.

Goal: Decrease processed foods:

- Pick one day during the week to cook up a couple forms of grain and flavor them yourself. I.e. – brown rice with garlic and basil or quinoa with chopped sundried tomatoes and parsley.
- Make your own soups.
- Pack leftovers for lunch rather than eating premade meals.
- Make sandwiches without processed sandwich meats (sliced chicken breast, egg salad, leftover meatloaf slices, or all veggies).

Get out your goal tracker sheet and add a specific goal that you think will be most beneficial to you. Then do whatever shopping or cooking you need to do to be sure you can easily attain this goal. Remember, keep the goal small. Any activity you do, will contribute to your long-term health!

Note:

If you feel you currently eat a healthy amount of grains (including whole grains), a healthy amount of proteins and few processed foods, consider mixing things up by trying something new! Try a new grain, try new recipes etc. Get creative with these food items.

■ Week #7: Fitness - Resistance is Futile

(Sorry about the dorky title...I couldn't resist) This week, we take another look at our fitness "routine". I say routine in quotes because many of us don't have an actual routine, and that isn't necessarily a bad thing...but we'll get to that soon.

In week 2 we talked about just getting ourselves moving. Walking, stretching, biking...just to increase our overall activity levels a little bit. This week, we are going to talk specifically about resistance training.

As we age and become more sedentary, our bodies begin to lose muscle mass. There are several reasons why we want to slow down or reverse this process. Increasing (or maintaining) our muscle mass keeps us strong and toned. Because women generally start off with less muscle mass, it doesn't take much loss before we notice the difference in our ability to use stairs or to lift objects. Having healthy muscle mass also helps us burn more calories, helping us to maintain a healthy weight. Resistance exercises build muscle mass, as well as maintain bone density – which is important for avoiding the negative affect of osteoporosis (which is not just a woman's disease).

So what exactly are resistance exercises? They are exercises that use weight (resistance) to build muscle strength. The weight can be dumbbells, ankle weights, jugs of water or your own body weight.

Here are a few common exercises that you can consider adding to your daily activities: Do several repetitions of these exercises.

Shrugs – holding weight in your hands, raise your shoulders.

Tricep extensions – holding light weights behind head with elbow by your ears pointing toward the ceiling; straighten the arm to lift the weight overhead.

Bicep curls – holding weights by your sides, bend your arms to life weights toward your shoulders/chest.

Pushups – On your knees, hands under yours shoulder, back straight; lower your body toward the floor maintaining a straight back.

Crunches – Similar to a sit-up, but rather than raising your whole body up to meet your knees, you only lift your shoulders up, keeping your chin off your chest. Think of lifting your shoulders up toward the ceiling and concentrate on using your abdominal muscles to do this.

Bridge – Lay on your back with your knees bent so your feet are close to your body. Push through your feet, using your hamstrings and gluts to lift your hips up off the floor.

Squats – stand with your feet hip width apart. Lower your body down as if you are preparing to sit in a chair, then use your thighs to lift yourself back up again. Repeat this several times. Focus on keeping your knees over your ankles. It is wise to keep a chair under you so you don't squat too low, which is not good for the knees.

Toe raises – Standing (holding a wall or chair for balance if needed), raise up on your toes, then lower. Keep your weight toward your big toe.

If you don't understand my description of any of these movements, or to double check how you should best align your body during the movements, you can find information on the web or at the library. Either will provide you detailed instructions on how to properly perform the exercise. Also, your cable network may have channels devoted to exercise and physical fitness. If you have any medical conditions, check with your doctor and /or physical therapist before doing resistance exercises.

These few exercises listed above will work most of the main muscles of your body. Of course there are probably a hundred other resistance exercises that will work these muscles and others. Feel free to do others...these are simply some suggestions.

The average person, just wanting to maintain decent muscle mass, should use intermediate amount of weights for their strength level (meaning that 8-12 reps is tiring, but after a few moments of rest you can do another 8-12 reps). If you find the muscles are incredibly sore the next day, you know you pushed it a little too hard and need to back off on the weights. Typically, after resistance work, it is best to let the muscles rest a day or two before working those muscles again. Some people do this by alternating muscle groups daily, or doing all muscle groups just 2-3 times a week. If you are just doing minimal reps with light weights, you could probably do the exercises daily.

The important thing is to push your body a little, but not too much. Listen to your body and start very slowly.

What exactly am I proposing for this week? Obviously, adding resistance exercises to your "routine". Now why do I keep putting the word routine in quotes? Because many of us get caught up in the idea that exercise is something that we must go do. That we have to carve out a big chunk of time from our schedules to do our exercise "routine"...whatever that may be. This is not true. When we talked about adding more movement into our day in week 2, I didn't say you had to commit to 30 minutes on the treadmill, right? Just 5 minutes of walking here, parking further away, going for an evening walk with your spouse etc. is all you needed to get moving. The same is true for resistance exercises. You don't have to go to the gym. You may find it helpful to have a set or two of dumbbells, but really even that isn't necessary. You can easily take two empty gallon jugs and add enough water to them so that they are a weight you feel is appropriate (One gallon of water weighs about 8 pounds). Then just add some of these exercises into your day. Often these can be done while you are doing something else. I often do squats while blow drying my hair and toe raises anytime I find myself standing in line somewhere. I do bicep curls right before getting dressed and crunches while watching TV. You get the idea here, right? Just start adding these exercises in throughout your day. Getting rid of the idea of an exercise routine often helps get rid of the excuses for avoiding exercise (i.e. "I don't have enough time").

Let's recap our changes. While several have been small daily changes, a couple were meant to be "one and done" or once in a while items.

- We are finding ways to add an additional serving of vegetables into our daily diet.
- We are sneaking exercise into our day (walking, stretching, and playing).
- We are finding a few minutes each day to be mindful, sit in silence and breathe.
- We have made a change that has decreased our chemical exposure.
- We have done something to support a charity or person in need.
- We are finding ways to add whole grains, limit processed foods or choose healthier proteins.
- We are finding ways to add resistance exercises into our week.

There are a lot of changes here, but if you have set small goals to move you in the right direction, it shouldn't be overwhelming. If you are feeling overwhelmed by these changes, you have a couple of options. Review your goals and consider if you bit off too much by making/setting a goal that was too much.

Remember, baby-steps. There is no sense in making goals that are too large to keep up with. If you need to, scale back on a couple of the goals you set.

Another option is to slow down. Maybe take two weeks (or more) for every change...allowing the change to really become a normal occurrence before moving on to add another. 90 days was just a suggestion...if it takes you longer, it takes you longer. The important thing is that the changes stick, not how fast you can get through the process.

So this week, set a goal to add some resistance exercises into your day.

Some ideas for resistance exercise:

- Do squats while you brush your teeth or blow dry your hair.
- Do 10 pushups before you get dressed in the morning.
- Do 10 bicep curls as soon as you get home in the evening.
- Do toe raises while waiting in line at the grocery store.
- Do crunches or triceps while watching TV in the evening.

Note:

If you routinely do resistance training, consider trying a new exercise to spice it up and get your body out of the exercise rut.

■ Week #8: Stimulate the Mind

I would like to start this chapter a little differently. I would like to take a moment to do a little exercise. Yes, I need you to really do it....don't just read about it and move on. Do it with me, please. It will only take a few minutes, but it is important to do it before you move on with the chapter. Get a piece of paper and a pen or open up a blank word document on your computer. Now imagine you are sitting on a plane for a long flight and the person next to you strikes up a conversation. They turn to you and say, "It looks like we are going to be here for a while; we might as well get to know each other...tell me about yourself." Now write out your answer...remember you have a long flight ahead, nowhere else to go and no one else to talk to...so you have all the time in the world, no need to rush. Write it all out....go ahead, I'll wait.

****

****

****

****

You're done already? Okay, read what you wrote and think about it for a minute. Did you talk about what interests you? What types of books you read or what your favorite color is? Did you talk about how you used to paint when you were younger or how you always wanted to write a book? Did you discuss your passion for music or your interest in French cooking? Did you talk about what you learned about yourself at the last empowerment seminar you attended or how you just ran your first 5k?

Or, did you talk about your job, your spouse, your kids, the town you live in, where you are flying too, where you grew up, how many siblings you have, etc. Did you talk about the roles you play in life or did you talk about you? This can be an eye opening exercise for people, as we realize we may have forgotten a bit of who we really are...what makes us tick...what makes us light up with excitement!

I find that often, we get so busy taking care of our responsibilities, that we get stuck in the monotony of everyday life. We forget to do things we enjoy or things that allow us to grow. We often spend so much time working, cleaning, repairing, parenting, providing, and nurturing that we don't make the time to feed our own needs.

Are you guilty of this as well?

I am frequently surprised by how many people think their personal happiness and growth should not be their priority and that they would be selfish if they tried to make it so. However, if you don't take care of yourself, if you don't stimulate your mind and make time for things that you enjoy, you risk losing your sense of joy, and even your sense of self. I see this often in people. They identify so deeply with all of their roles in life, that they have forgotten who they are when they aren't a parent, a spouse, a homeowner, a friend, a sister, a son, an employee, etc...

We all tend to lose our sense of self to some degree at some point in our lives. In order to get out of our rut of identifying more with our roles than ourselves, I propose another exercise. This can be done as a journaling exercise, a meditation, or you could even talk it out with someone that will listen more and talk less. No matter which method you think will work best for you, I suggest you start by closing your eyes, taking 3 – 4 deep breaths in and out...relaxing the body and calming the mind. As you exhale, feel yourself become centered and connected with your true essence. Ask yourself who you are when nobody is watching...when you are all alone. Not at home, but outside of the comfort zone called your daily routine. If you woke up tomorrow in a new town, surrounded by new people....when they introduce themselves to you, who would they meet? Sit with that question for a minute and then either open your eyes to talk or write, or keep your eyes shut and meditate on that thought. The focus here is on what brings you joy, what interests you, what excites you. If your immediate answer is my job, my kids or my spouse bring me joy, than look deeper. What brings you joy when they aren't there?

This can be a very difficult exercise if you are very separated from your sense of self. If that is the case, do not despair. Repeat this exercise several times, think about what you enjoyed in the past....do you have a hobby that you used to enjoy but no longer participate in because you are pulled to do other things instead? Or maybe there are interests that crossed your mind but you just never followed up on.... Is there a class you would like to take but don't because you just don't have the time? Is there a book you would love to read but you don't want to waste time sitting around doing nothing? When was the last time you went out dancing or anything else that was just for fun?

As we "grow up", we often forget who we are and what we enjoy. We lose ourselves to our roles in life.

This week is all about finding some time do something that stimulates your mind and excites your soul. It is important to routinely do things that we enjoy, things that bring joy to our lives and that when missing, leave us depressed and just a shell of who we could be. Life is short, make it how you want it, right?

Study after study show that getting lost in an activity that we love and enjoy, significantly increases our level of happiness. Positive psychologists call this "flow". Feeling fulfilled and joyful requires spending some time in the flow...doing what brings you joy. Have you ever been busy in the garden, planning a project, working on a craft, building or painting, or anything really...only to find that you completely lost track of time. You were just so "into" what you were doing that you didn't realize you missed a meal or that hours had passed? When that happened, you were "in the flow".

You may realize, as you sit down to create this goal, that even after doing the exercises above, you still don't know what you like to do anymore or what you might even be interested in learning! So start with what you know or just try something new. I'm not suggesting you run out and enroll in college to get your Master's degree in basket weaving.... I'm suggesting you think for a moment about something you used to do when you were younger and start there.

Ideas:

-   You used to love art class? Grab a pencil and a sketch pad or stop at an art store for some paint.
-   You used to read mystery novels? Stop by the library and pick up a new release.
-   You played guitar? Tune it up and play.
-   You used to whip up gourmet meals before the kids came along? You used to love building things out of wood? You loved helping your Grandmother in the garden? You used to jog or play baseball?

See how you can reconnect with one of these interests.

Still completely void of inspiration?

-   Ask your friends or co-workers what they like to do.
-   Check out the community education sessions near you to see if anything sounds remotely interesting.
-   Find a park nearby and just get out in nature for a bit and see if you can find some inspiration there.
-   Turn on the radio or checkout an online radio player such as Pandora and search down music that you like.
-   Go online and take an aptitude test to see what might interest you.

Once you have decided on what you are interested in trying, you have 2 tasks to accomplish this week. First, is to obtain any supplies you might need. You may need to schedule a trip to a store or library; or find the time to rummage through the basement or garage, etc. The second task is even more important; you need to set aside the time to actually do this joyful activity! This is where people fall down on this goal, the follow through. It doesn't have to be a big time commitment, just enough to accomplish your goal. Schedule it in your calendar and keep it!

Now, let me be honest here. Depending on your interest, this might be a lot to spring on you and expect you to follow through with in just one week's time. If you have to register for a class, get a lot of supplies or schedule a significant amount of time, one week may simply not be enough time. I understand this, and I don't wish to stress you out by asking you to do the impossible. So start with what you can, schedule what you need to, and be sure to follow through! Just be sure you do something toward your goal of feeding your mind and bringing excitement and joy into your life, because this week's task is of the utmost importance in bringing you real happiness!!!!

Note:

If you already spend time each week working on a hobby or doing something that leaves you feeling fulfilled and joyful, then consider spending this week repeating and delving deeper into a topic from a previous week.

■ Week #9: Tea, Water & Herbal Remedies

As you may be noticing, I am trying to keep a certain level of variety in the changes we are making together. Holistic Wellness involves so many aspects of life that variety is easy! My hope is that not only does this variety keep you interested, but that it will also help prevent you from becoming overwhelmed with changes.

As we enter month three, I want to reiterate the importance of making your changes small! Baby steps are the most successful!! If you find that you are feeling overwhelmed with change, you can do one of two things: 1) reevaluate the size of your changes and reset any goal that you now realize is too big, making it a more manageable goal or 2) take a week off. I don't mean to quit the changes you have already started, but to simply take a week of no new changes. This sometimes just allows us to get a better grasp on the changes we have started, allowing them to become our new normal, before continuing on.

So now that you are ready to move ahead with yet another change, let's talk Tea, Water, and Herbal Remedies.

This is one of the few times I will say that you may want to consider adding two new goals to this week, because they will be rather simple. However, if that sounds like too much, then don't. You know yourself best. Do what feels right for you!

Let's start with the topic of water. Many of us drink way too little water and walk around in a constant state of mild dehydration. Even a slight amount of dehydration can cause many health issues, such as headaches, decreased immunity, dry skin, fatigue and inability to concentrate. Dehydration can also cause you to overeat as the brain tries to get you to ingest more liquids by telling your body you are hungry.

When it comes to dehydration, water is not the only answer. Fluids in any form help, except alcoholic and caffeinated beverages (okay, they help a little but since they have diuretic affects, the benefit is minimized). But while fruit juice or even soup may cure dehydration, they do this while also adding calories. Many drinks that we turn to routinely, like soda, sweetened teas, fancy coffee drinks, etc., contain empty calories (meaning no other nutritional benefit)....so because of this, water is indeed the drink of choice.

There are many recommendations and calculations regarding how many ounces of water you should consume a day. Often you will hear 8 glasses (64oz) a day for the average person. This is a great place to start. If you are very active, take certain drugs or your doctor has suggested you need more than this, then, by all means, drink more than 64 oz. But if tracking ounces is too much for you, simply use the p-gauge. What is that you ask? It's simple, really. When you use the restroom, simply note the color of your urine. If it is the color of diluted lemonade, you are probably getting plenty of water. If it is darker in color, you probably require more. Keep in mind that vitamins and certain drugs may color your urine and make this gauge inappropriate.

Now, let us move on to the subject of tea. This is one of my favorites. There is so much to say about tea, but I will try to keep it simple. Tea comes in so many varieties that it is impossible to list them all: Black teas (such as Earl Grey), Green teas (such as Jasmine), Red teas (such as Rooibos), White teas and many versions in-between. But as a rule, almost any tea you choose will have a benefit to you. Teas are known for their high levels of antioxidants. Many reports have suggested that Green tea in particular, helps to prevent some types of cancer. While this may or may not be true, I think most experts agree that increasing antioxidants is a good thing for your body's immune response. Herbal teas also provide benefits specific to the herbs they include and are usually naturally free of caffeine. If the tea you drink does not contain caffeine, it is naturally flavored water and therefore counts toward your daily water intake.

The subject of teas and herbal remedies are closely related. This is because one of the most common ways to use herbs is via tea. One of my all-time favorite herbs/teas is Chamomile. I often tell people, if you are going to add 1 herb to your "diet", make it Chamomile. In a perfect world, we would drink chamomile tea every day. This herb is a wonderful nervine tonic herb – which means drinking it often, helps our body deal with day to day stresses that come our way. It is also wonderful for digestion and easing tension...and it tastes great too!

Speaking of herbal remedies, the best place to look is in your own kitchen. Here are a few things you will find there and how to use them:

Garlic

- Raw for antibacterial, antiviral properties. Mince it into salad dressing, mustard or honey to add raw garlic into your food. This is great anytime you feel a cold coming on or even before it gets that far.
- Cooked garlic is great for your cardiovascular health. Cook with it often to keep your heart healthy.

Lemon

- Added to water it provides a refreshing drink that also helps alkalinize your body. Since we often eat very acidic foods, this is a great tonic for the body.

Vinegar

- Combine with an equal part honey, to ease a cough.
- Dilute with hot water to create a steam to relieve cough and congestion.

Oregano

- Make a steam with dried or fresh oregano and hot water. This is great for inflamed sinuses.

Lavender

- Add dried lavender to chamomile tea for a relaxing evening blend.
- Add lavender tea to your bath water for relaxation.
- Use a good essential oil to ease muscle tension and stress headaches.

Mint

- Mint tea soothes the belly and eases headaches. (Avoid peppermint if you suffer from acid reflux)

Calendula

- You can use the dried herb in your bath water to soothe scrapes and burns, or find natural burn salves made with this herb.

Chamomile

- Rinsing hair with a dilute chamomile tea is moisturizing and is especially nice when used on blonde hair.

The options here are almost endless. You can stick with dried herbs/teas, use capsules or try essential oils. I must caution you to be sure you get any herbs/products from reputable companies and I especially warn you to be careful with essential oils. Many 100% pure oils are still poison when ingested and are meant for aromatherapy only (and do you really even want to breathe that?). Look for oil brands that are okay to be taken internally...such as DoTerra or Young Living.

You may want to look into trying some more unusual herbs, such as:

VALERIAN for tension headaches, **PASSIONFLOWER** for insomnia, **GINGER** for stomach upset, **ECHINACEA** for cold & flu, **GINSENG** or **ASTRAGALUS** for fatigue or **NETTLES** for iron deficiency. Many of these herbs can be found in capsule form in herbal or natural stores. However, discuss any issues with your doctor, as relatively minor symptoms could indicate a more serious condition.

Now that we have discussed the importance of water, tea and herbal remedies please take a moment and think of what change(s) you want to make this week.

Again, this may be an easy week to add 2 small changes...but do only what you are comfortable with.

Here are some suggestions:

-   Start your day with 8 oz of room temperature water with the juice of ¼ lemon.

- Exchange one sugary/alcoholic/caffeinated drink for water every day.
- Exchange one cup of coffee for one cup of green tea.
- Start a bedtime routine of unwinding with a cup of Chamomile tea.
- Drink a cup of herbal mint tea after dinner.
- Drink 3- 8 Oz. glasses (of water throughout the morning, to be finished before lunch.
- Replace sleeping pills such as Tylenol PM with Passionflower capsules.
- Drink tea with your lunch.
- Make a lavender bath part of your normal weekend activities.
- Add fresh garlic into your normal cooking regimen.

These are all very simple ideas, yes? Now get out your goal tracker sheet and document what exactly you intend to do this week.

Note:

If you already drink plenty of water, you love tea and your medicine cabinet is full of herbal remedies, then consider either trying something new (a new remedy or a new tea), or consider spending this week repeating and delving deeper into a topic from a previous week.

■ Week #10: Friends & Family

How often do you spend real quality time with close friends and family members? If you are anything like me (and so many others), you may find that you are so busy with all of your daily responsibilities that you struggle to find time to connect with friends...or, you find that loved ones whom you used to be so close with, have drifted away. In this day and age, it is so easy to connect with those we love, but yet we often feel more isolated than ever.

There are several reasons for this. First, we seem to equate busy-ness with success. In doing this, we create an internal environment that tells us we are not successful if we happen to have plenty of downtime. Second, in this day and age, we easily get lost in a sea of technology...isolated in a world that is supposed to help us stay connected. We have traded phone calls for texts, family dinners for Facebook updates, and going out with friends for sitting home with our smartphones. It is no wonder we often feel disconnected and isolated.

Can you see a bit of yourself in any of those words? If so, this week is just what you need. Many of us feel that after a long day of work, what we need is a little down time on the couch with our TV, smartphone or tablet. While downtime is important, this type of downtime is often mind-numbing and is not fulfilling to your soul. Try something for yourself...Take a moment and remember how you felt after the last time you had a real conversation with someone you care about. This could be a close friend or a close relative. Think for a moment about how you felt after that conversation. Now think of your last Facebook interaction, and think for a moment about how you felt after that? Is there a difference? Most people notice a large difference....feeling fulfilled and happy after the real conversation and feeling at best, indifferent after the online interactions. This is very similar to the discussions we had in weeks 5 & 8. Interaction with people feeds your mind and soul in the same ways service work, learning and hobbies do. Not only are relationships fulfilling on a normal given day....but in a time of tragedy or struggle, having a close network to turn to can be a lifesaver (or at the very least, a sanity-saver).

Relationships are what life is all about. Unfortunately we live in a society that often prioritizes things over people. I think it's time to change that and I think you will agree. This week we are going to focus on making some meaningful connections with people that are important to us.

This week, in addition to all of the other great changes we have made, we will in some way, connect with a person with whom we have (or used to have) a close connection. The more personal this interaction is, the better. Face to face is the goal, but if you haven't seen a person in a long time, a phone call or even a text or Facebook message may be the best you can do to start reconnecting. Just know that your goal is to work toward a real time connection with someone close.

Ideas:

- Set up a lunch date with an old (or new) friend.
- Call a sibling.
- Arrange a family get-together (such as a simple potluck picnic).
- Host a dinner party for old college buddies.
- Start a new family tradition that involves spending time together.
- Set a reminder on your phone for every Sunday evening to "phone a friend".

What if you don't have many friends or family? Try these ideas to meet new people and start creating your circle:

- Join a meet-up group. These are clubs you can find online to meet people in your area with similar interests.
- Schedule a happy hour with coworkers.
- Host a "mommy (or daddy) and me" play group with your child's school-mates.
- Join a gym and get to know people there.
- Check out your local library for book clubs.
- Sign up for an adult learning class at your local school/college to meet people.

The goal for this week is to connect with people. What this means for you will vary greatly depending on how social you currently are and how much you have let personal relationships slide. In order to do this, pick one of these items to try this week. You can choose something that is fairly simple and easy for you, or if you know you really lack in this area, you may be inspired to try something big. In the end, you know what will do the most for you...so do what will give you the best outcome!

■ Week #11: Sleep

This week our goal is just one simple word....sleep. During sleep, our mind processes all that has happened during the day while our bodies rejuvenate and heal. Without adequate sleep, we get sick and find that our minds don't function as well as they should. This is obviously an oversimplification of why we must sleep, but I think it's enough to understand the importance of sleep to our bodies.

Many of us don't get an adequate amount of sleep every night. This can be because we are so busy we don't feel we have time. It could be that we are prioritizing other things over sleep (TV, Facebook, cleaning), or it could be that we are just stressed and anxious to the point where even though we go to bed, we just can't quiet our mind enough to sleep.

Let's look at each of these reasons separately...

"I'm just so busy I can't devote 8 hours a day to sleep." Really? Just like exercise, "too busy" is seldom a valid excuse for not getting enough sleep. We make time for the things we prioritize. And often, the things we actually prioritize in our lives are not the things that are really important to us. I don't know why so many of us are guilty of this, but we are. If I had to map out my perfect day (one that would be healthy, peaceful, enjoyable and enriching), it would not include TV, gossip, Facebook, or many other similar time wasters. Yet I often find myself giving up much of my daily time to these things. Why? Often I think it's just lack of awareness. If I don't consider what my priorities are, I can easily just get lost in the void and miss out on what does matter.

At this time, I'm going to ask you to do an exercise. Map out a typical day. It might be good to do a week day and a weekend day to capture the variety. Then map out your perfect day (also one week day, one weekend day). For your perfect day, remember to envision a life that is healthy, peaceful, enjoyable and enriching. If you are overwhelmed right now, you may think your perfect day would just be lying on the couch all day long, but that is just the fatigue talking. You wouldn't find a life of doing nothing but lying on the couch fulfilling, would you? So think of how you would really want to live your daily life...think about the goals you have already set for yourself over the last several weeks. You have been setting these goals to get you closer to a place of holistic wellness...where you are balancing all aspects of yourself to live a healthy and happy life. I would therefore expect your perfect day would include many (if not all) of these new changes like eating nourishing food, doing something to promote a healthy active body, time with friends or family, learning or doing something interesting. As part of taking care and feeling your best, I bet it also includes a good night's sleep or maybe a nap. Looking at the disconnects between the two schedules (perfect vs actual), can teach you a lot about yourself, but right now, what we are focusing on is sleep. Is there anything on your actual schedule that is not on your perfect schedule, that you could give up to allow more time for sleep? Maybe you could pack your lunch while cleaning up from dinner to allow yourself to sleep in 15 minutes in the morning. Maybe you can give up some TV or other timewasters? Be honest, because most people do indeed find that when they look at their actual day, they wasted a lot of time doing things they didn't really care about, or spent time with people they don't even like.

Now, if you are occasionally choosing something fulfilling over sleep, that's okay. I occasionally stay up too late because I'm hanging out with friends, teaching a late class or attending a class myself. This is fine (better than fine actually), as long as it is something you enjoy, and not happening so often that you suffer from sleep deprivation.

What about the times when you leave yourself plenty of time for sleep, but you just can't get to sleep? Insomnia can affect us all, occasionally. Learning to let go of anxiety and allow your mind and body to calm can be difficult for some. If you have persistent insomnia, talk to your doctor to be sure there isn't a medical reason behind it.

If your insomnia is just occasional or your doctor has ruled out a medical condition, here are a few ideas that can help:

- Create a bedtime routine that is soothing and relaxing.
- Turn off TV and other electronics one hour before bed to allow your mind to quiet down.
- Relax with an herbal soother such as chamomile and lavender tea or tea with sleepy herbs such as valerian and passionflower.
- Meditate, in the morning and as part of your bedtime routine.
- Once in bed, do a progressive relaxation. Starting with your toes toward your head, focus to relax one body part at a time (feet, ankles, calves thighs......neck, jaw, scalp, and forehead)
- Try a breathing exercise, such as 4,2,8,2...inhale in a count of 4, hold your breath for a count of 2, control and slow your exhale for a count of 8, hold for 2. Controlling and slowing your exhale calms your body and slows your heart.

- Spray a mist of water and lavender essential oil on your pillow before bed.
- Avoid caffeine after 3:00pm (or earlier if it really affects you).
- Enjoy a relaxing bath with lavender oil, candles, dimmed lights and peaceful music.
- Remove the TV or other distractions from your bedroom. The bedroom should be used for sleep and lovemaking... that's it. This trains your brain that bed = sleep.
- If you find that you still can't calm your mind, journaling may be just the ticket. Journaling allows you to process your worries, thoughts, plans etc. You process your thoughts and get them out of your head and onto paper. Sitting with a notebook and a pen, writing out your thoughts is therapeutic and meditative. It allows your brain to let go of your thoughts and relax.

The goal this week is to ensure you are getting adequate sleep. Look over the suggestions above and choose a specific action that will help ensure you are getting enough shut-eye. Write your goal on your tracker form and make this change!

Note:

If you consistently get 8+ hours of good sleep, then consider spending this week repeating and delving deeper into a topic from a previous week.

■ Week #12: Spirituality, Religion, Nature

This is our last official week, so what shall we discuss?

So often we get so caught up in the petty details of our life that we lose sight of the bigger picture. There is a duality that we must realize: we are just a drop in the ocean, miniscule in the grand scheme of the universe, and at the same time, our actions affect the world. Sometimes our affect is direct, other times we inspire or influence actions (or inaction) in others. Keeping this in mind, let's spend some time focusing inward and outward.

This week we focus on our sense of spirituality and connection with nature. For some this may include your religious beliefs, but you do not need to belong to a religious order to feel a sense of connection to something greater than you. Let's connect to our sense of humility, our faith that we are part of something greater than us, that we are not the center of the universe and that our actions affect the rest of the world.

Connecting with nature, taking time to nurture our religious beliefs and explore our spirituality are perfect ways to end our first round of life changes to bring ourselves closer to living from a place of holistic wellness. How do we do this? Some of these ideas may be reminiscent of some suggestions made earlier in the book. Choose something that speaks to you, add it to your goal list and allow yourself to shine!!

Here are a few ideas, but feel free to think outside the box and do something that speaks directly to your spiritual side:

- Start a journal to get in touch with your thoughts and feelings.
- Meditate daily.
- Read a book on Buddhism or one by a spiritual leader of your liking.
- Find a church in your area to join (or rejoin).

- Visit a local park or take a walk in some neighboring woods.
- Find a local charity to support.
- Pray.
- Start a gratitude journal to remind yourself of all the good in the world.
- Look around your home and find ways you could live a little greener.
  - use cloth napkins
  - substitute chemical cleaners with vinegar
  - use energy saving light bulbs and appliances
  - donate extra items to charity
  - lower your heat settings, raise your A/C temperature setting
- Take a walk and pick up litter on your way.
- Observe wildlife in your area.

This week is all about realizing you are divine and connected to everything around you. Treat yourself, and the world, with love and respect.

◼ Week #13: Extra Assignment

All of the changes you have made over the last three months are great! You have made great changes toward improving your health and well-being. However, there may be some personal care that you have been neglecting. Now that you have made some substantial improvements in your lifestyle you should be feeling pretty good about yourself.

Therefore, now is the perfect time to make any appointments and take care of things you have been procrastinating about. Below is a list of commonly avoided items, but everyone is different. This week, take care of something you have been putting off.

Common procrastinations:

- Dentist appointment
- Mammogram
- Colonoscopy
- Prostate exam and blood work
- Annual physical
- Drafting a will
- Health care proxy and living will
- Discussing final wishes with aging parents
- Household maintenance (cleaning gutters, checking furnace, cleaning chimney)
- Changing batteries in smoke detectors
- Making a budget or meeting with a financial advisor

What have you been putting off? Do it this week. Not only is there likely a benefit for completing the task itself, but there is also mental relief at finally doing something you have been avoiding.

Or, you may have a vice that you would like to kick...but as you recall, I advised against addressing vices at the beginning of this book. However, now you have made 12 positive changes... it might be time for you to seriously look at stopping a vice. If you're a smoker, consider creating a plan to slowly decrease the number of cigarettes you smoke. If you feel you drink too much, start decreasing the number of daily drinks. If you sleep around or gamble, consider a plan to eradicate these behaviors. Just remember what we talked about 3 months ago. Success is MUCH more likely if you can limit negative reinforcement and find a way to create positive reinforcements.

Choose your goal for this week, add it to your list and just do it.

■ Parting Thoughts

Congratulations!!!! You did it! You should feel so proud. You have made huge strides to creating a healthy, happy and fulfilling lifestyle for yourself. If you really followed through with the changes, you are feeling the difference. However, since the changes you made were all small, the benefits may have snuck up on you. Take a moment to revisit all the changes you made for yourself. Acknowledge the hard work and how these changes have accumulated to create a big shift in how you take care of yourself and how you live your life. Are you proud of yourself? You should be!!!

If you started the process already in a pretty good place, you might be done. The past 3 months may have been just enough to help you reach your goals. If that is the case, I'm very happy for you! Keep up the good work and enjoy your happy and healthy lifestyle. It will serve you well!

However, for many of us, three months is not enough time to get us from where we were to where we want to be. If that is the case for you, you will find that the last three months have brought about great changes, but you don't quite feel like you are living in the manner that you really want. You might feel better, but you aren't quite ready to describe your lifestyle as healthy and fulfilling. For those of you in this situation, I have a very simple answer for you....turn back to page one and start again. Continue to build on the changes you already made, add more positive changes to continue on your path toward the lifestyle that you want to live...toward feeling the way you want to feel.

You may choose to skip over some of the chapters on your second and third time through, but do yourself a favor and don't dismiss them out of hand. Reread the chapters and truly consider if there is further growth you can obtain from each and every chapter. If there continues to be one chapter that really feels necessary to you, feel free to stick with that chapter for more than one week. This is your journey...do what you need to get to where you want to be!

One last thought...sometimes our loved ones feel insecure, jealous or confused by our desire to better ourselves. Don't let any naysayers in your life discourage you from making changes that will make your life better. Don't let peer pressure convince you to forego your fruits and veggies for fast food, or to stop your meditation practice because it sounds too hippy-ish! This is your life...live it in a manner that is healthy, happy, balanced and fulfilling....live it from a place of HOLISTIC WELLNESS!!!!!

For further growth and development, visit my website www.holisticwellnesswithtracy.com and *like* my facebook page https://www.facebook.com/holisticwellnesswithtracy

Use the tools listed in the appendix and let my website and facebook page continue to inspire you!

I look forward to supporting you on your journey!!!

■ Appendix List

Tools you may want to use as you implement changes.

Appendix 1: **90 Days Goal List**. Feel free to print up a few copies to write in. Use to keep track of the goals you set.

Appendix 2: **Food Tracker**. Use this to make a true assessment of your eating habits and periodically check how you're doing.

Appendix 3: **Meal Planning Shopping List**. Use this form to plan out weekly meals & snacks and to create your shopping list.

Appendix 4: **Goal Tracker**. Allows you to keep track of meeting your goals day by day.

These tools can be found on a private page within my website:

http://www.holisticwellnesswithtracy.com/90-days-to-holistic-wellness-goal-list.html

Week 1: _____
(adding 1 extra daily serving to my normal diet)

Week 2: _____
(adding 10 minutes of exercise into my daily activity)

Week 3: _____
(meditating, even just 1-2 minutes a day)

Week 4: _____
(reducing chemical exposure)

Week 5: _____
(support a charity or do good deeds)

Week 6: _____
(diet tweak – add wh.grain, better protein, less processed food)

Week 7: _____
(adding resistance exercise)

Week 8: _____
(do something you enjoy, learn something new)

Week 9: _____
(tea, water, herbs)

Week 10: _____
(connect with friends/family)

Week 11: _____
(sleep)

Week 12: _____
(spirituality, religion, nature)

Week 13: _____

Food Group Tracker

As you eat, X off servings   (X=full serving; / = half serving)

| | minimum recommended serving |
| | recommended servings |

Holistic Wellness with Tracy

Bread/Cereal/Grains

6-11 servings (1/2 of which should be whole grain)

1 slice of bread, 1 cup cold cereal,

1/2 bagel, 1/2 cup rice or cooked cereal

Vegetables

3-5 servings

1 cup cooked or raw veg, 2 cups greens

1 cup vegetable soup or juice

Fruits

2-4 servings

1 medium piece of fruit, 1/2 grapefruit

8 oz 100% juice, 1/2 cup dried fruit

Meat/Fish/Protein

2-3 servings

2-3 oz meat, fish, poultry

1/4 cup beans, 1 TBSP nut bitter, 1 egg

Dairy

2-4 servings

1 cup milk (dairy or other), 1.5 oz cheese

6-8oz yogurt

Oil

sparingly

1 TBSP oil, margarine, butter, salad dressing

Sweets, Alcohol

keep to a minimum

Chips, Soda, Alcoholic drinks, Candy, Cookies, Cakes

See individual labels to determine serving size

Water

some say 8 glasses a day. Another rule of thumb is 1/2 oz for every lb you weigh.

Meal/Shopping Planner   www.holisticwellnesswithtracy.com

Date		Date	
Breakfast:		Breakfast:	
Snack:		Snack:	
Lunch:		Lunch:	
Snack:		Snack:	
Dinner:		Dinner:	

Date		Date	
Breakfast:		Breakfast:	
Snack:		Snack:	
Lunch:		Lunch:	
Snack:		Snack:	
Dinner:		Dinner:	

Date		Date	
Breakfast:		Breakfast:	
Snack:		Snack:	
Lunch:		Lunch:	
Snack:		Snack:	
Dinner:		Dinner:	

SHOPPING LIST

Daily Goal Tracker

GOAL / DAY	1	2	3	4	5	6	7	8	9	10	11	12	13	14	15	16	17	18	19	20	21	22	23	24	25	26	27	28	29	30	31

■ About the Author

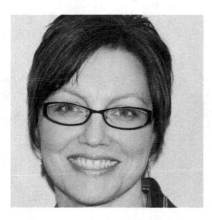

Tracy Martorana, owner of Holistic Wellness with Tracy and Tracy's Teas, is a nutrition & wellness consultant, herbalist, and meditation instructor. She inspires her clients to make changes in their daily habits to create the fulfilling life they desire. Tracy lives with her husband and daughter in a small town outside of Rochester, New York.

Printed in the United States
By Bookmasters